THE HIDDENURSE™

THE HIDDENURSE™

HOW TO BECOME A PUBLIC HEALTH NURSE

Latronda Davis, MPH, RN, BSN

Davis, Latronda

    The Hiddenurse™: How to become a Public Health Nurse / Latronda Davis / Non-Fiction / Medical / Nursing

ISBN: 978-1-7374565-0-6

Cover design: Ebony Rose
Editor: Shaundale Johnson

Request for information and/or Hosting/Speaking Engagements: Please contact me at latrondadavis@gmail.com or visit my website at www.hiddenurse.com.

Dedication

This is dedicated to all the nurses in the world, especially to my underrated nurses in public health.

Acknowledgments

To God, thank you for transforming my life, covering me when I didn't know I needed the protection, giving provision over my life, and allowing me to do the best I can to follow in the footsteps of Jesus, in my passion and purpose in life.

To my mom, Terrie Davis, you are my superhero. Your kindness, joy, and optimistic outlook has gotten me to a place in life where I know no fear. I admire your beauty and grace, which has been the most powerful inspiration in my life. I love you with all my heart.

To my dad, my angel, Timothy Davis, you will forever be the man arms I will run into. You always made me feel like I can have anything in the world and assured me that life will work out just like how I wanted. Though I truly miss your physical presence, I know you are in heaven smiling down on me and cracking jokes with the Lord.

To my brother, Adonis Davis, you made me proud to be a big sister. I love watching you as you continue to grow and mature into the man you have become and are becoming. You taught me how to step out of my comfort zone and try new endeavors.

To the rest of my family and friends, thank you for your continued love and support. You all are my tribe. Thanks for being my biggest fans!!

Thank you to everyone who strives to grow and help others grow. The world is a better place thanks to people who want to serve and lead others in love.

Contents

Introduction

~Why I Do What I Do and Love What I Do

Many nurses fall into public health, unknowingly. Most don't go into nursing wanting to do public health. In fact, I didn't even plan to go into nursing.

The first day of my biology freshman class, the professor asked us to raise our hands if we wanted to become medical doctors. Of course, most of the class raised their hands (including me, who wanted to become a gynecologist) because that's why most students choose to become biology majors in the first place. Then she proceeded to give the most profound revelation ever, in my opinion, which was "All of you will not become medical doctors. And there is more to biology than just being a doctor." That statement alone, helped me to open my eyes to other possibilities in healthcare. Needless to say, I switched majors after my freshman year. This did not throw me off track, and I was still able to graduate in four years and could have done so in 3½. *Just a tip for college in general: If you ever want to finish faster, attend summer school.*

My journey into public health nursing started back in the summer of 2006 while in undergrad, the summer before my junior year. My major was health care management at this point. I applied for a paid internship called Project Imhotep and was accepted to participate as an intern. Project Imhotep is established through a partnership between Morehouse College and the Centers for Disease Control and Prevention (CDC). If you would like to find out more information or apply to this internship, please use the following link, https://www.morehouse.edu/academics/centers-and-institutes/public-health-sciences-institute/project-imhotep/).

During the summer of 2006, I was placed at Clayton County Board of Health for my internship. My work included maternal and child health research and assisting in the Men's Health Clinic. During my senior year of college, I did my senior practicum at the Southwest Georgia Health District. My project centered around sexually transmitted diseases/infections (STDs/STIs) and the Human Immunodeficiency Virus (HIV) education and promotion. What I learned from these experiences was that servitude, compassion, and care for everyone's quality of life are skills you must naturally possess to be fulfilled in these roles. Having a natural heart to care for people (which is why I wanted to become a doctor in the first place) also comes with being a servant first. Serving God and his people, along with having the God-given purpose to care for the overall health of others, public health seemed to be very divine and in alignment with what I should have been doing all along.

I graduated at the worst time—in 2008 when the recession hit. I thought about staying in school, becoming a dual major and getting my nursing degree then. However, I was not in the right mind set at the time, so I returned home and decided to go to graduate school instead. Now, when I wanted to become a doctor, I always desired to attend Morehouse School of Medicine (MSM) for medical school, but I never thought I would have been attending for graduate school. I wanted to attend Emory University for graduate school.

In Fall of 2009, I started graduate school at MSM as a full-time student along with working a full-time job. (Thank you, God, for 6:00 pm classes.) My concentration was Health Administration, Management and Policy (HAMP). During graduate school, I had to complete a practicum requirement and thesis. I did my practicum at the Environmental Protection Agency (EPA). I served as a graduate research fellow in the Office of Superfund Public Affairs and Community Outreach. After I graduated in 2011, I was accepted into the Directors of Health Promotion and Education Internship as a Centers for Disease Control and Prevention (CDC) Guest Researcher. I was placed in the community at a community-based organization (CBO) called STAND, Inc. They ended up hiring me on full-time as the Assistant Project Coordinator/Case-Coach Manager after my fellowship ended. My work catered to coordinating services surrounding recidivism (repeat offender) for 16-24-year old's who had been involved with the criminal justice system. Unfortunately, that was a two-year funded grant position, so at about month 22, I ended up receiving a position at Clayton County Board of Health (which is where my first public health work experience started at in 2006 with my undergrad internship) as the ARTAS HIV Testing/Linkage Coordinator.

Side Note: I stayed on as a contractor to finish out the work for the last 2 months of the grant. I would go into STAND, Inc. (the community-based organization I worked for) office a few days a week after work. I was doing a lot, but I made it work for me lol.

It's so surreal how things come back full circle in your life. This is when I decided to go back to nursing school so that I could push my public health career forward. So, I intentionally went into nursing knowing I was going back into public health. Now the only school I applied to was...drum roll please, Emory University (who knew). I got accepted contingent upon me finishing my pre-requisites, which I completed during the spring and summer semesters of 2014 before starting in August of 2014. I will not bore you with life in nursing school, as it is another chapter that goes into more detail; however, I graduated in May of 2016, and I only wanted to do two years at the bedside. God and I had an honest conversation about me working only two years in the hospital and going right back into public health before I entered nursing school, and that's exactly what I did.

In August of 2016, I started working at the Veterans Affairs Medical Center (VAMC) in a one-year post Baccalaureate Nurse Residency Program on an oncology medical surgical floor. Concurrently, I worked part-time as a registered nurse (RN) at a plastic surgery center. I later went on to work at Northside hospital for one year on the clinical observation unit/cardiac floor. This floor served as an overflow unit for our Cardiac Care Unit (CCU). In August of 2018, I was back in public health and haven't looked back since.

***Disclaimer:** Public health nursing is not a field you go into if you are looking to make lots of money (stay at the bedside for that lol). It's a field you choose because you have a servant's heart, and you truly care about the quality of life for others.*

Chapter 1
What is Public Health Nursing?

~Defining Public Health Nursing

S o, let's start off with a few definitions. I know you all are wondering what Public Health Nursing is! You are probably like, *Nursing, yeah, I know what that is. Public Health, maybe not so much.*

Let's first define nursing. "Nursing encompasses autonomous and collaborative care of individuals of all ages, families, groups and communities, sick or well and in all settings. Nursing includes the promotion of health, prevention of illness, and the care of ill, disabled and dying people. Advocacy, promotion of a safe environment, research, participation in shaping health policy and in patient and health systems management, and education are also key nursing roles (International Council of Nurses, 2002)". In simpler terms, nursing is using care and education to help people reach their optimal physical and mental health state through all facets of life.

Health is defined as a "state of complete physical, mental and social well-being and not merely the absence of disease or infirmity (World Health Organization (WHO), 1946)." In simpler terms, health goes beyond just the physical. It truly takes a holistic approach when addressing the lives of individuals. Public Health is "the science and art of preventing disease, prolonging life, and promoting health through the organized efforts and informed choices of society, organizations, public and private communities, and individuals (Winslow, 1920)." In simpler terms, public health is everything. It's in every aspect of our lives.

Now let's put all the terms together, and you get Public Health Nursing. Public Health Nursing is "the practice of promoting and protecting the health of populations using knowledge from nursing, social, and public health sciences. Public health nursing practice focuses on population health, with the goal of promoting health, and preventing disease and disability (American Public Health Association, Public Health Nursing Section, 2013)." So, a public health nurse is basically a nurse who chooses to work in a "traditional" public health setting. Traditional settings include health departments, state or local and agencies such as the Center for Disease Control and Prevention (CDC). I say "traditional" because most healthcare settings such as hospitals/clinics, education systems, pharmacies, transportation agencies, food industry, etc. are not necessarily classified as public health settings.

As stated previously, because public health is essentially in everything, these particular settings will fall under what we call in public health, the social determinants of health. The social determinants of health "are conditions in the environments in which people are born, live, learn, work, play, worship, and age that affect a wide range of health, functioning, and quality-of-life outcomes and risks (Office of Disease Prevention and Health Promotion, 2020)". This simply means that conditions such as economic standings and social influences impact your quality of life, along with your physical surroundings such as schools, green spaces, and workplaces.

Recent 21st century pandemics have made us very aware of how important public health is and how it impacts our daily lives. There are laws that help govern public health and how it is implemented throughout the world. Particularly, in the United States, we have police powers. Public health police powers allow states to authorize and enforce health, isolation and quarantine, and inspection of laws to prevent the spread of disease (Galva et al, 2005). This means in the event of a natural disaster, pandemic, epidemic, etc. (basically, things out of our control that affects the entire population general well-being), the interest in community protection is placed before the individual person. Though it is secondary, the health and autonomy of the individual is protected to the best extent possible in these circumstances.

A great example of this is tuberculosis or TB. Within public health, individuals do not have sole control over their treatment when the disease is a threat to the community (Richards and Rathbun, 1999). A TB infected individual does not have the right to refuse diagnosis or treatment and remain free to spread the disease. If this happens, which is very rare, this person will have to remain isolated for the rest of lives unless they agree to treatment.

With all that said, you may be wondering:

1. Why should I become a public health nurse?
2. How do I become a public health nurse?
3. What are some tips on becoming successful at public health nursing?

These next four mini chapters will cover those questions and provide you with practical tips and advice, that will help you to carry out a nursing (regardless of whatever specialty you choose) and public health career path.

Something to consider: We must respect that Public Health Nursing is a specialty just like any other field of nursing. Public health nurses are vital to the world. We are not just nurses who are here in times of crisis, but we are protecting, preventing, and promoting every day to improve your quality of life in every way.

Chapter 2
Why Should I Become a Public Health Nurse?

~Because you already are one!

Well, I hate to break this to you. *No, I really don't hate it, lol; I actually love to tell nurses this.* But essentially when you decide to become a nurse, pass boards, and receive those official letters RN (LPN for some) behind your name, you have officially signed up to be a public health nurse. There will more than likely be a point in your career when you may be pulled to assist in public health emergencies, volunteer at a health fair, or you may, on your own desires want to do medical missions trips in the summer. But trust me, there will come a time, where you will have to step outside the typical hospital setting and into the community or other parts of the world. This will happen by choice or obligation.

So, why do you want to become a public health nurse? 1) your technically already one (sort of lol) and 2) public health nurses have endless opportunities to help and care for the world. Some of the opportunities include working for local, state, or federal government agencies, community-based organizations (CBOs), non-profit associations such as American Cancer Society and the list goes on. Sounds fun, right?

Nursing, in general, allows you to create your own lane, in my opinion. If you choose to venture into the public health route, then you open your mind to different ideas and career paths that bridge treatment (traditional medical system) and prevention (public health) together. Ultimately, making you the best fit for anything in the realm of health (as defined by WHO, so remember health is holistic) and healthcare.

What do we contribute to the world? Public health nurses contribute to every aspect of the world from a single person, a family, the community, or systems (government, health system, law enforcement, school systems, etc.), with the goal of keeping people healthy in healthy communities. If you are interested in learning more about how we keep communities healthy, please visit this website to learn more, https://purposebuiltcommunities.org.

Public health nurses provide a wide range of skills along with the ability to connect the public to systems that are vital to their health. Some of these skills include disease surveillance, health education and promotion, policy development, conducting needs assessments, outreach and referral, and health and disease investigation. Education and promotion are two of the main ways public health nurses contribute. Here are a few ways we contribute:

- Demonstrate safety practices such as seat belt safety, car seat safety, and elderly safety
- Teach family members how to care for sick loved ones
- Encourage testing and screening for diseases

- Encourage vaccination against diseases
- Teach prenatal and baby care
- Promote wellness and improved quality of life
- Advocate for safer and healthier neighborhoods

Fun Facts about Public Health Contributions in General:

- Controlled infectious diseases through sanitation (yes, trash pickup) and hygiene (yes, handwashing)
- Encouraged vaccinations to reduce diseases such as smallpox and measles
- Contributed to safer workplaces
- Improved car safety (seat belt laws were one of the first major public health laws to be passed)
- Enhanced family planning efforts through affordable birth control options and pre-natal care
- Performed food safety checks (please check your restaurant ratings before sitting down to eat)
- Added fluoridation in our local tap water to reduce dental decay

- Used health education campaigns that promoted tobacco cessation (which means to stop), which led to a reduction in tobacco use throughout the country
- To learn more, visit Ten Great Public Health Achievements -- United States, 1900-1999 (cdc.gov)

Recent Public Health Initiatives in 2020:

- Medicaid Expansion
- Paid medical and family sick leave
- Taxes for public education and public transit
- Minimum wage increases (24 states)
- Voter enfranchisement
- Decriminalization on low-level drug possession
- Police oversight boards
- To learn more, visit

  https://www.networkforphl.org/

Chapter 3

How Do I Become a Public Health nurse?

~Choose a path, earn a degree, and get your license!

I n this chapter, I am going to give you practical steps and applications to become a public health nurse. This section will be broken into three groups: high school/college/non-traditional students, individuals already in the nursing field, and individuals with other degrees who may or may not have experience in public health.

For high school/college/non-traditional students:

Decide. Think about what your major will be in college; whether you want to go into nursing, public health or become a dual major. Also, you may want to look into a two-year nursing program (Associate Degree), though I highly recommend as well as the Institute of Medicine (IOM) to pursue a four-year Bachelor of Science in Nursing (BSN) degree. *Apply, get in, and start.* Most four-year BSN programs require pre-requisite classes and an entrance exam (typically, the Test for Academic Skills (TEAS)) to be accepted into the school's nursing program. If you need assistance with TEAS, please visit, https://atitesting.com/teas/study-manual. Make sure you speak with your college advisor to discuss the prerequisite classes you need to take. It's nothing worse than taking and paying for unnecessary classes that are NOT needed for your major or required for you to graduate.

Volunteer. Local health fairs, health departments, and CBOs are great places to volunteer at along with schools, food banks, nursing homes, etc. Volunteering and providing service is the groundwork for public health. I believe it helps build the character of a public health nurse and it is what makes us stand out from all other nursing specialties.

Become an Intern. Internships, fellowships, and externships are your best friend when it comes to exploring the field of public health or any field, in general. The hands-on experience and knowledge you gain, gives you a deeper perspective on if this field is the right fit for you. If you are interested in any public health internship or fellowship , please follow this link to view opportunities available for everyone from high school to doctoral students, https://www.cdc.gov/fellowships/short-term/index.html.

Study, Study, and Study. Nursing school is not for the faint of heart. So, there will be a lot of sacrifice. Be prepared to miss out on some events but still allow yourself to have fun and enjoy the college experience. Just DO NOT neglect your studying. Come up with a study plan to assist you in staying on task.

Travel. While in college, take advantage of opportunities that may provide global travel for healthcare. Global health is a big proponent of public health. A lot of public health threats occur across our borders, so it gives you a chance to learn how public health and healthcare looks in other countries. It also doesn't hurt that you get to see new places and add to your life experiences. I would suggest you go to your global health department at your school and seek out available opportunities. These academic departments are normally located within the school of public health, nursing, medicine, or possibly foreign affairs.

Participate in school. If your school has a public health nursing course as a part of the curriculum (some schools don't), take advantage of that class and the learning opportunities presented such as the emergency preparedness simulations drills. Join different groups or clubs that are geared towards public health and community service. If it is possible, for your senior clinical hours or rotation, see if you can choose a place that is not in the traditional hospital setting. I did mine at Kaiser Permanente, in their Gastroenterology (GI) clinic. My school considered this to be a "community rotation." Out of about 120 students, only two of us wanted to do a community rotation. This equates to 0.016% of the nursing students, not even close to 1%. You might as well say 0%. This is how scarce public health nurses are in the real world. They are few and far between.

Take and PASS the test. The last step is to graduate and pass the National Council Licensure Examination (NCLEX) to become a Registered Nurse (RN)! My tips for NCLEX would be:

1. Remember the basics from nursing school such as normal and abnormal lab value ranges, dosage calculations, infection precautions/control, personal protection equipment (PPE) measures, Marlow's hierarchy of need, and your ABCs (airway, breathing, circulation).
2. Use Saunders NCLEX prep book.
3. Consider using UWorld, which is an online study tool. I did the 30-day option and felt very comfortable when I went to take my exam. This site mimics the look of NCLEX, so it makes you very comfortable

with the test. Personally, the questions were much harder on here than NCLEX. Please visit UWorld at, https://nursing.uworld.com/nclex-rn/?_ga=2.4615478.449660058.1617302881-1360630110.1617302880.

4. Study by body system. Focusing on one system at a time can prevent you from becoming overwhelmed or overloaded with different information.

5. Practice at least 75 different questions a day in one sitting. You need to build up your stamina to answering these types of questions in a reasonable timeframe. 75 questions to me, are enough questions in a day to practice and review the answers and rationales. Treat studying for NCLEX like a job; and lastly,

6. Take advantage of the free prep your school may have. All of it will work in your favor to pass! And remember to *remain calm;* it's just a test. Whether you pass at 75 questions or 250 questions, you are a registered nurse (RN). If you

fail, it's not the end of the world. Study again, remain calm, and repeat the test until you pass. Since you have experienced taking the test before, you will be comfortable with the format so that should work in your favor the next time around.

Pray. Another major step (really it is the first step) is to pray, fast and meditate. I cannot stress the importance of how having a spiritual life (whatever faith you practice) to help ground and motivate you during this time will be vital to your survival in nursing school. I would bring my daily devotional bible to school every day and read it before or after class. Getting up for 8:00 am classes and trying to beat Atlanta traffic did not leave me with enough time to pray, meditate, and read in the morning. As I was not getting up any earlier than I already had too, lol. These practices were already a part of my daily life before nursing school, so they truly continued to help me stay positive and as stress-free as I could possibly be lol.

Take care of your health. Having consistent spiritual practices also help your emotional and mental health during school as well as in life. If you need additional support such as a counselor or therapist, please don't hesitate to use one. A lot of my classmates had mental health breakdowns, so the stress is REAL. Also, don't forget about your physical health. Continue to incorporate small breaks for exercise and eat as healthy as you possibly can. Make sure to bring your lunch, dinner, or healthy snacks with you while on campus or wherever you will spend most of your time studying. *Don't overload on caffeine trying to study all night!*

Side Note: I passed NCLEX with 75 questions in about an hour. My friend (also a nurse) would probably say less than an hour because I called her going in and immediately after I came out, and she was surprised (but not really lol) because it was so quick for me. We had literally just gotten off the phone. But I am also a quick test taker because either I know the answer, or I don't. I don't dwell on questions. And I would advise you not to either because the test shuts off at 250 questions. This means if it has not shut off at 75, you are still in the game to pass, and you have up to 5 hours to take it. If it shuts off at 75, either you did extremely well or extremely bad. So, don't fret; be glad if you do get past 75 because you still have a chance.

Fun Fact: *NCSBN statistics show it takes first-time, United States-educated test-takers just over two hours to take the RN exam and answer an average of 120 questions. Please visit https://www.ncsbn.org for more information on NCLEX.*

For those of you who are already nurses, you have two choices, from my experience:

Note: *This section is truly for individuals who are nurses with no public health experience or limited public health experience. If you have an associates in nursing, I advise completing a RN to BSN program, if you plan on obtaining a Masters in any field but it's not required.*

1) The 1st option is to obtain a job in public health such as at the local health departments, non-profit organizations, federal or state public health agencies (ex. Environmental Protection Agency (EPA), Centers for Disease Control and Prevention (CDC), Food and Drug Administration (FDA), Occupational Safety and Health Administration (OSHA), etc.). You will be able to gain knowledge and experience at the same time. Now, the downside to this option is that it could be challenging obtaining one of these positions without previous public health work experience or having an advanced degree in public health or similar

field. Nevertheless, it's definitely a viable option.

2) The 2nd option is going back to obtain a Master's in Public Health (MPH). I would suggest applying to a program where you must be a full-time student, preferably in person. The traditional setting for public health will afford you a lot more opportunities, experiences, a vast network, and resources, in my opinion. Online options are good for convenience and affordability.

With a public health degree, you now have the basic knowledge and training to go into the public health field. Since you typically must do a practicum and a thesis, if your program requires it (mine certainly did, shoutout to Morehouse School of Medicine), you would have gained public health work experience, research experience, and who knows, you may even come out with a publication. See my first publication at https://muse.jhu.edu/article/380424/pdf.

As you can see, obtaining a job will be easier than the second option. Now the downside to this second option is that it takes some time, which is at least two years, and some money. Still, it is a highly viable option. So just choose what best suits your needs.

For individuals who have other non-nursing degrees and who may or may not have public health experience:

This last section is about the route I took. It's for those who already went to undergrad (obtained any other degree besides a BSN) and/or who also may have already obtained a Master's in Public Health (MPH) or another masters. The only option you have, my dear, is to go back to school. Fortunately, they have a lot of accelerated BSN programs for individuals with a previous bachelor's degree. An associate degree program is still an option also, but the time commitment may be the same. With either one, you will have to check with the school you are considering and their prerequisite requirements. Please take the classes if you have not taken them in your previous undergraduate program.

Tip: Check to make sure your credits will still transfer because the universities and/or colleges will not take them after a certain number of years have passed (generally after 7 years).

This process does take time and cost money. I was able to work full-time, attend my pre-requisite classes in the evening time, online, and Saturday mornings at two different schools. I paid for those classes out of pocket to fulfill those requirements. Most schools will accept you contingent upon you completing the pre-requisites. And again, the process after you are in nursing school is just the same as mentioned in the high school/college/non-traditional student section.

The accelerated programs only take two years because you have already completed those fundamental classes within your first degree and completed pre-requisites, so you go right into the nursing program. Now, your experience will be different since you are coming from a different background or public health, so you will be gaining nursing experience and skills. Once you are done, it is highly recommended that you complete a two-year residency in the hospital to develop and sharpen those fundamental nursing clinical skills. Many jobs will not hire you without at least two years of "clinical" experience (which typically refers to hospital experience). Then, you can venture into public health. However, there is a shift in public health where some local health departments are starting to take newly graduated nurses. In fact, some health departments are starting public health nurse residency programs. Soon, there will be potential in obtaining a public health nursing job as a new graduate.

Chapter 4

Where Do You Find Jobs/Career Opportunities?

~WORK, WORK, WORK (in my Rihanna voice)

Well, the good news is that public health jobs are plentiful, if you open your mind and eyes to all the possibilities that surround you daily. Now I am going to say it again, public health nursing is not for those who expect a big paycheck. Public Health, in general, is a very underfunded field, though it contributes so much to society's wellbeing. *It's sad, I know*! The most common opportunities would be your local county health departments, health districts, state health department, Centers for Disease Control and Prevention (CDC), and U.S Department of Health and Human Services (HHS). Other common agencies would be the Environmental Protection Agency (EPA), Food and Drug Administration (FDA), Occupational Safety and Health Administration (OSHA), National Institute of Occupational Safety and Health (NIOSH), and National Institutes of Health (NIH). Now your non-traditional opportunities would be community-based organizations and health associations such as American Heart Association, American Lung Association, American Cancer Society, etc. Health associations are perfect for those of us who have a passion for certain health conditions; giving you the ability to just focus on that area. Becoming a professor at a public health school is also another great opportunity. Hospitals also have non-clinical roles that public health nurses can serve in. These last two type of opportunities will require you to keep your eyes open, and on the hunt, because they go fast. To get started on your search, here are a few links you can use to find opportunities now:

1. https://apps.sph.emory.edu/PHEC/
2. https://www.usajobs.gov/
3. https://heart.jobs/?utm_campaign=heart.org-Footer&vs=2896&utm_medium=Other&utm_sou rce=heart.org-Footer
4. https://www.lung.org/about-us/careers

You are not limited to these links or associations. Typically, individuals use these specific sites because they are the most popular. These are here to get you started on your career search. Make sure to search for areas that are of a particular interest to you. Google will become your best friend if it's not already!

Opportunities for Growth – *Learning Never Stops*!

There are always opportunities for growth, and we should always be looking for them. There are certifications you can obtain while working as a bedside nurse in your area such as Medical-Surgical Nursing Certification, Critical Care Nursing Certification, and Emergency Room

Nursing Certification. You can participate in training opportunities that are of interest to you. For example, you may work in Labor and Delivery, but you have an interest in cosmetics. You can attend a laser hair removal training and become certified in that cosmetic procedure. Look for training opportunities your job may offer for free. *Also, check your work email on a regular basis so you won't miss out on those free opportunities.*

Publications are another great opportunity, if you have a heart for research, work in research, or work on certain projects or programs. Always look for opportunities to publish. I would suggest before you start a new project, think about the information that could come out of it. Publications allow us to put the data out, so that we can see what is working and what is not. It also helps to build evidence-based practices, so that we all are practicing and providing the same standard of care. Another opportunity is to become a nurse entrepreneur. You can start your own scrub line, write for medical and public health magazines, be a consultant, etc. The sky's the limit when it comes to creating your own business.

In closing, I hope this book provided insightful tips on how to become a public health nurse. If anything, I wanted to provide tangible resources to refer to once you finished reading. I wish you well on whatever journey you choose to take in life, and I hope it brings you many blessings, love, joy, peace, and happiness. As this book ends, I leave you with this quote, "*The most valuable possession you can own is an open heart. The most powerful weapon you can be is an instrument of peace.*" - Carlos Santana

References and Links

1. International Council of Nurses. (2002). Nursing Definitions. Available at https://www.icn.ch/nursing-policy/nursing-definitions.
2. World Health Organization (WHO). (1946). Definition of health. Preamble to the Constitution of the World Health Organization as adopted by the International Health Conference. WHO, Geneva. Available at Constitution (who.int).
3. Winslow, Charles-Edward A. (1920) The untilled fields of public health. Science 51 (1306):23-33. Available at THE UNTILLED FIELDS OF PUBLIC HEALTH | Science (sciencemag.org).
4. American Public Health Association, Public Health Nursing Section. (2013). The definition and practice of public health nursing: A statement of the public health nursing section. Washington, DC: American Public Health Association. Available at https://www.apha.org/~/media/files/pdf/membergroups/phn/nursingdefinition.ashx.

5. Office of Disease Prevention and Health Promotion. (2020). Social Determinants of Health. Available at https://www.healthypeople.gov/2020/topics-objectives/topic/social-determinants-of-health.

6. Galva, J. E., Atchison, C., & Levey, S. (2005). Public health strategy and the police powers of the state. Public health reports (Washington, D.C.: 1974), 120 Suppl 1(Suppl 1), 20–27. Available at https://doi.org/10.1177/00333549051200S106

7. Richards III, E. & Rathbun, K. (1999). The Role of the Police Power in 21st Century Public Health. Editorial. Sexually Transmitted Diseases Volume 26, No. 6. Available at https://biotech.law.lsu.edu/cphl/articles/pp-jstd.pdf.

8. https://www.morehouse.edu/academics/centers-and-institutes/public-health-sciences-institute/project-imhotep/

9. https://purposebuiltcommunities.org

10. Ten Great Public Health Achievements -- United States, 1900-1999 (cdc.gov)

11. https://www.networkforphl.org/

12. https://nursing.uworld.com/nclex-rn/?_ga=2.4615478.449660058.1617302881-1360630110.1617302880

13. https://apps.sph.emory.edu/PHEC/

14. https://www.usajobs.gov/

15. https://heart.jobs/?utm_campaign=heart.org-Footer&vs=2896&utm_medium=Other&utm_source=heart.org-Footer

16. https://www.lung.org/about-us/careers

17. https://muse.jhu.edu/article/380424/pdf

About the Author

Latronda Davis, MPH, RN, BSN is a native of East Point, GA and currently serves as a Nurse Program Manager in Chronic Disease at the Georgia Department of Public Health. With a combined 10+ years of public health and nursing experience, she is committed to improving the health of individuals and building healthier communities. Her area of expertise includes chronic disease management and prevention, HIV, grant writing, and project management.

She previously served as the Assistant Coordinator for a youth-focused project (STAND, Inc.), where she facilitated a court-ordered domestic violence invention program, specialized in substance abuse treatment, HIV/AIDS prevention, and Re-Entry for a few years. She then went on to become the HIV Linkage Coordinator at Clayton County Board of Health, where she was responsible for designing, implementing, and maintaining procedures to improve the overall quality of HIV linkage services for the underserved. She loves and is committed to what she does because she is able to promote holistic health, protect and prolong life, and prevent illnesses.

Latronda's nursing experiences includes the Atlanta VA hospital, where she worked as a staff RN on an Oncology-medical/surgical unit for patients receiving chemotherapy as well Northside Hospital as a Cardiac RN on the clinical observation unit for patients with an extensive cardiac history. Additionally, she worked for a plastic surgery center doing pre, intra, and post-op care. She obtained her Bachelor of Science in Healthcare Management from Albany State University. She obtained her Master's in Public Health with a concentration in Health Administration, Management, and Policy from Morehouse School of Medicine. Then pursued a Bachelor of Science in Nursing from Emory University Nell Hodgson School of Nursing.

She is the owner/founder of The HIDDENURSE™, LLC., which provides tutoring for college and high school students, scholarships, coaching services for individuals interested in pursuing nursing and/or public health and additional nursing and public health consulting services.